TODAY...

- **4,000** CHILDREN WILL BE KILLED BY DIARRHOEA

- **1,400** WOMEN WILL DIE NEEDLESSLY IN PREGNANCY OR CHILD-BIRTH

- **80 MILLION** SCHOOL-AGE CHILDREN, MOST OF THEM GIRLS, WILL NOT GO TO SCHOOL

- **37,000** PEOPLE WILL DIE OF INFECTIOUS DISEASES

Introduction

Classrooms with teachers, clinics with nurses, affordable medicines, running taps, and working toilets – for millions of people in poor countries these things are a distant dream, and there is no reason why this should be the case. Yet these vital public services – health, education, water and sanitation – can transform the lives of poor people. They make society more equal. They are the key to making poverty history.

Building strong public services for all is hardly a new idea: it is the foundation upon which many of today's rich countries are built. More recently, developing countries have followed suit, with impressive results. Botswana, Sri Lanka, Malaysia, Uganda, and Kerala state in India, for example, have within a generation made advances in health and education that took industrialised countries 200 years to achieve.

Building strong public services works. Poor countries must invest in free health, education, water and sanitation. And they should be given the money and power to do so.

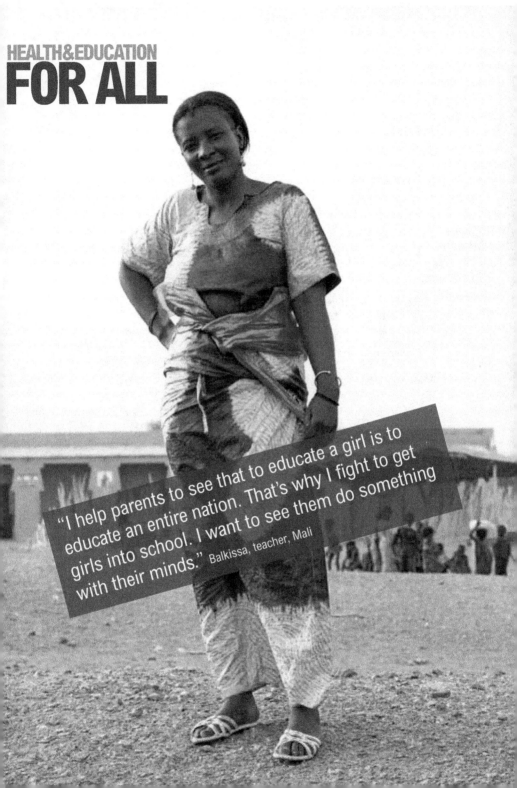

HEALTH&EDUCATION
FOR ALL

"I help parents to see that to educate a girl is to educate an entire nation. That's why I fight to get girls into school. I want to see them do something with their minds." Balkissa, teacher, Mali

Contents

This is Afsana. She's a teacher at Kassmandi Khund School in rural India.

Afsana was a pupil at the school where she now teaches. In a big break from local convention, she left her village to study for a teaching degree in a nearby city. "The girls I teach tell me they're motivated by me," she says. "They think if I can leave the village, study at university, and become a teacher, then they can too."

She grew up living with her parents, five sisters, and four brothers. Her parents – both tailors – played a big part in her becoming a teacher. "They managed somehow to find the money so I could finish high school, and help me study to become a teacher."

Traditionally, educating girls has been considered less important here than educating boys. As Afsana explains, before she got her degree, none of the local girls used to leave the village and continue their studies. Now, many do, and more and more parents are starting to see the value of education.

The Indian government's commitment to education has improved a lot recently, she says. Teachers' salaries and training are better than they were, and more is being spent on books and teaching materials. As a result, parents – especially those with girls – are now more inclined to send their children to school.

Afsana loves working with children, especially "interacting with them and helping them learn," but conditions here aren't easy. Afsana is one of two teachers at the school, and each of them has to teach around 175 children. As she says: "The children have different levels of learning, so how can the quality be as good as it needs to be?"

Imagine what she could achieve if there were more teachers and she could spend a little more time with her students.

INDIA PROFILE

- 836 million people in India are poor and vulnerable. Compare this with India's 33 billionaires; the largest number in Asia, including Japan.
- Of all the countries in the world, India has the largest number of people without access to education.
- More than half of all Indian women are illiterate.
- Maternal and infant mortality rates in the country's poorest states are worse than in sub-Saharan Africa.

**ONE PERSON CAN MAKE A BIG DIFFERENCE.
IMAGINE WHAT SIX MILLION CAN DO.**

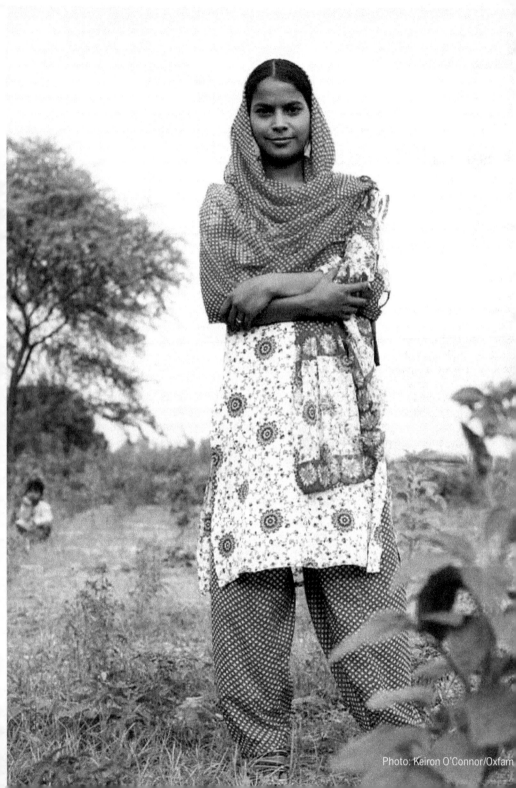

What needs to happen

Poor-country governments

Governments must take responsibility
for providing quality essential services:
- that are accessible to all their citizens
  – including women, girls, and the
  very poorest
- that are free of charge (water should
  be subsidised for poor people)
- that are well-staffed by trained and
  motivated teachers, doctors, and nurses
  on regular decent salaries
- that provide appropriate and affordable
  medicines: free of charge or priced within
  all patients' reach.

There are no short cuts to governments
expanding their provision of services –
providing classrooms, clinics, and clean
water, and training more teachers and health
workers. Civil-society organisations and
private companies can make important
contributions, but they must be properly
regulated and integrated into strong public
systems, and not seen as substitutes
for them.

While some governments have made great
strides, too many lack the cash, the capacity,
or the commitment to act.

Rich-country governments and international institutions

Rich countries and international financial
institutions such as the World Bank need
to play their role too.

They need to:
- stop pushing private-sector initiatives
  that do not benefit poor people, and
  support proven public-sector
  solutions instead
- keep their promise to give 0.7 per cent of
  their national income as foreign aid and
  allocate at least 20 per cent of that aid to
  essential services
- provide more long-term, predictable aid,
  which is channelled through government
  budgets, so that countries are able to plan
  and invest in good quality health and
  education
- extend debt cancellation to all countries
  that are unable to reach the Millennium
  Development Goals (MDGs) under their
  debt burden.

In addition, rich countries and
pharmaceutical companies need to:
- stop imposing higher intellectual property
  protection, which deprives poor people of
  vital medicines.

PROVIDING LONG-TERM, PREDICTABLE AID IS EASILY AFFORDABLE.

TO MEET THE MDGS ON HEALTH, EDUCATION, AND WATER AND SANITATION WOULD REQUIRE AN EXTRA $47 BILLION A YEAR. ANNUAL GLOBAL MILITARY SPENDING IS $1 TRILLION.

Public successes

Sri Lanka: less income than Kazakhstan, but with a healthier population and more children in school.

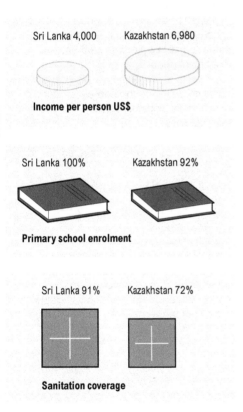

Sri Lanka 4,000   Kazakhstan 6,980

Income per person US$

Sri Lanka 100%   Kazakhstan 92%

Primary school enrolment

Sri Lanka 91%   Kazakhstan 72%

Sanitation coverage

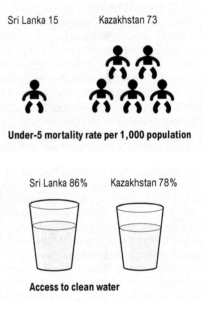

Sri Lanka 15   Kazakhstan 73

Under-5 mortality rate per 1,000 population

Sri Lanka 86%   Kazakhstan 78%

Access to clean water

Sources: Income per person: GNI in purchasing power parity in international dollars, World Bank World Development Indicators Database 2004. Child survival: under-5 mortality rate per 1,000 population, 2003 data from UNICEF: www.childinfo.org/areas/childmortality/u5data.php. Schooling: net primary enrolment rate, 2002-03 data from UNDP: http://hdr.undp.org/statistics/data/indicators.cfm?x=117&y=1&z=1. Water: percentage of the population with access to improved drinking water, 2002 data from UNICEF: www.childinfo.org/areas/water/countrydata.php. Sanitation: percentage of population with sanitation, 2002 data from UNICEF: www.childinfo.org/areas/sanitation/countrydata.php

Governments that provide essential services for all

Oxfam's Essential Services Index assesses governments by ranking developing countries' performance in four social areas compared with their per person national income:
- child survival rates
- schooling
- access to safe water
- access to sanitation.

The Index shows that some governments have performed unexpectedly well: in **Sri Lanka**, even though more than 33 per cent of its population lives below the poverty line:
- maternal mortality rates are among the lowest in the world
- there is a 96 per cent chance a woman will be attended by a qualified midwife
- there is free medical treatment in public clinics, staffed by qualified nurses, within walking distance
- free primary schooling, and education for girls is free up to university level.

Compare this with **Kazakhstan**, where despite having 60 per cent more income per person, a child is nearly five times more likely to die in its first five years, and is far less likely to go to school, drink clean water, or have the use of a latrine.

Other successes include Uganda and Brazil – they have doubled the number of children in school, halved AIDS deaths, and extended safe water and sanitation to millions of people.

It shows that even the poorest countries can achieve huge amounts where there is the political will.

Successful governments have achieved results by:
- guaranteeing essential services available to all
- expanding government provision of services
- abolishing fees in health and education
- subsidising water and sanitation services
- expanding services into rural areas
- investing in teachers and health workers
- strengthening women's social status and autonomy as users and providers of services.

Where governments fail to act

"I serve 100–150 patients a week and they come to get treatment for TB, family planning, and diarrhoea. I come from this area and know the people here. I spend the average day worrrying because of financial hardship. I do not take fees from the patients. The primary reason for being a health worker
is to serve the people."
Beauty Mandal, health worker, Bangladesh

Despite successes, there are other poor countries where millions of people cannot afford to see a doctor, daughters have never been to school, and homes have neither taps nor toilets.

**Government inaction:
women and equality**

In Yemen, where government spending on essential services is low, the first to suffer are women.

In Yemen:
- a woman has only a one-in-three chance of being able to read and write
- a woman has only a one-in-five chance of being attended by a midwife
- a woman's child has a one-in-three chance of being malnourished
- a woman's child has a one-in-nine chance of dying before their fifth birthday
- if a woman lives in a rural area, her family is unlikely to be able to obtain medical care, clean water, or basic sanitation.

In fact, across the developing world, women:
- are more likely than men to fall ill, but less likely to receive medical care
- are expected to care for sick family members, but are often the last to be sent to school and the first to be taken out of school when money is short
- almost everywhere lose much of their day hauling buckets of water over long distances.

SERVICES ROUTINELY FAIL WOMEN AND GIRLS, YET INVESTING IN THEIR WELFARE IS THE CORNERSTONE OF DEVELOPMENT — INCREASING THEIR LIFE CHANCES AND THOSE OF THEIR CHILDREN.

This is Emilien. He's a doctor at the district hospital in Ansongo, Mali.

He's also something of a miracle worker. Despite having to deal with staff shortages, insufficient funding, a lack of water, and a sporadic electricity supply, since arriving at this rural hospital he's helped tackle some serious local health problems. "We've eradicated meningitis and whooping cough, and you can count the number of measles cases on one hand. I know change is possible – that's what gives me hope."

Emilien decided to be a doctor when he was a child. He trained in the capital, Bamako, but unlike most of the doctors who qualified with him, decided to work in rural Mali.

Ansongo is the main hospital for the region, and referrals come from 11 health centres. Staffing levels, however, are nowhere near adequate.

"There are two doctors, including myself. There are few nurses that are trained to the level needed. There aren't any doctors or nurses with specialist skills like radiography, and there's a problem finding obstetrician nurses to look after mothers and children."

Working in secluded villages also brings challenges. Many local people are pastoralists who move regularly. "To reach nomadic people you need to go to them, but we only have two cars and few trained staff."

Emilien is understandably proud of what has been achieved. "It's a sensational feeling to change the health of a village. It motivates me to work hard for the people, and inspires me to keep going."

Government support has increased recently. There is now no charge for Caesarian births, mosquito nets are freely available, anti-malarial tablets will soon be free for under-fives, and the price of medicines is falling.

But while Emilien still has to contend with many obstacles, the progress he has made seems incredible. "I am very proud to be a doctor and I love my job."

MALI PROFILE

- Mali has the highest percentage of people living below the poverty line of any country in the world. Ninety per cent of Malians survive on less than two dollars a day.
- One-in-four children die before they reach their fifth birthday.
- Eight out of ten women cannot read.

ONE PERSON CAN MAKE A BIG DIFFERENCE.
IMAGINE WHAT SIX MILLION CAN DO.

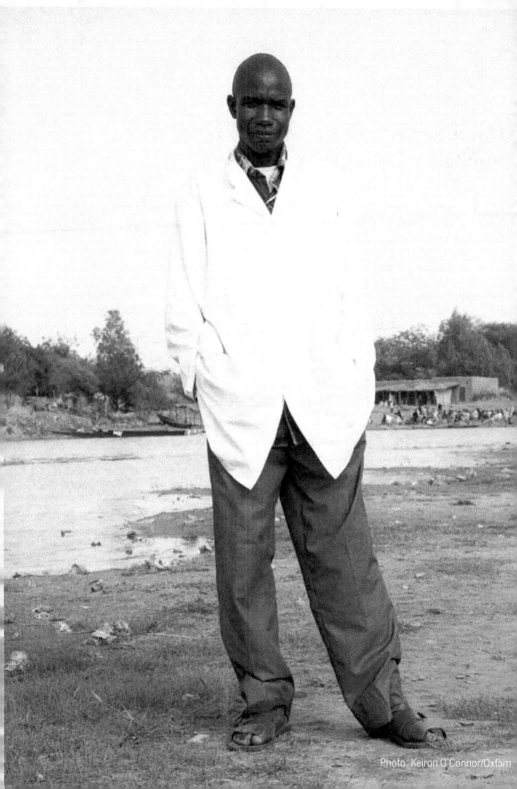

Public failures:
Fees – a life or death issue

"In the health centre they get annoyed when they treat you. If you don't have the money they won't take you. Then what? Well, you'll just be left to die."
Marta Maria Molina Aguilar, mother of a sick child, Nicaragua

For the vast majority of poor people in developing countries public services are:
- unavailable
- skewed towards the needs of the rich
- dauntingly expensive.

All of which drives up social inequality.

- Despite obvious gains in countries that have abolished fees in primary education, children still have to pay to go to school in 89 out of 103 developing countries. This forces many poor children to leave education – particularly girls.

- Most poor people have to pay for medicines. In some countries it can equate to 50–80 per cent of people's available income.

- In one district of Nigeria, the number of women dying in child-birth doubled after fees were introduced for maternal health services.

- In Georgia, the introduction of fees for health care saw hospital admission rates fall by 66 per cent.

- Deprived of public water services, poor consumers have to buy water from private traders, spending up to five times more per litre than richer consumers who have access to piped water.

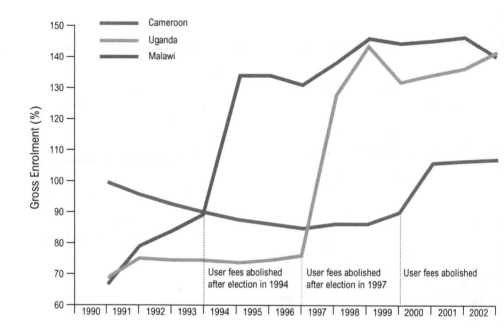

Abolishing school and health fees

Abolishing user fees for primary schooling and basic health care can have an immediate impact on the take-up of services. For water, which no-one can do without, the issue is not take-up but improving access for poor people and ensuring that a finite resource is shared equitably. Fees must then be structured to ensure that a minimum daily amount is free or affordable for poor people.

(Source: World Bank website: http://devdata.worldbank.org/edstats/query/default.htm)

Public failures:
Missing professionals

Globally, there are shortages of 1.9 million teachers and 4.25 million health workers.

Today, many governments lack the money and the workforce to build up public services to the scale and quality required.

The public services that do exist are kept afloat by a skeleton staff of poorly paid, overworked, and undervalued teachers and health workers – for example, teachers' salaries in least-developed countries have halved since 1970. These are the unsung heroes struggling to do their best in

crumbling public services. A government schoolteacher in Cameroon summed it up: "Becoming a teacher is like signing a contract with poverty."

Based on the Education for All target of one trained teacher for every 40 school-aged children:
- at least 30 countries do not have enough trained primary school teachers to educate their children
- in 11 of these countries, there are not enough teachers for more than half of the school-aged children.

Missing teachers

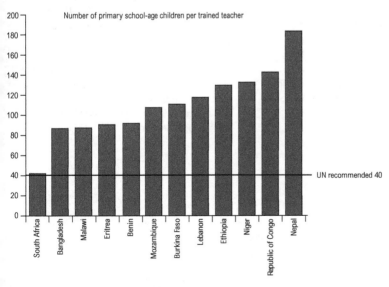

Number of primary school-age children per trained teacher

UN recommended 40

(Source: Oxfam calculations, data from UNESCO 2005)

Missing health workers

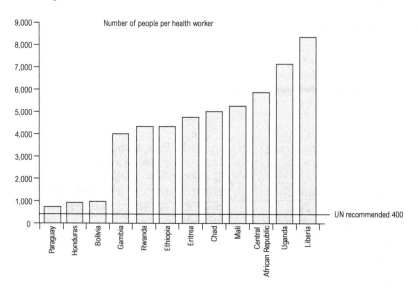

(Source: Oxfam calculations, based on data from Joint Learning Initiative 2004)

Based on a minimum standard of 2.5 health workers per 1,000 population:
- at least 75 countries do not have enough trained health workers to meet their needs
- of these, 53 countries have fewer than half of the trained health workers needed
- in ten countries, there are only enough trained health workers to cover ten per cent of the population.

HIV and AIDS redoubles the challenge – Africa is likely to lose 20 per cent of its health workers to the disease in the coming years. Moreover, many health workers are risking their lives because they have to work without gloves.

More than 40 million people are living with HIV and AIDS, and around 8,000 of them die every day as a result – mostly in the world's poorest countries.

"As much as we want to scale up, there are no people. You can't translate money into action when there are no people."
Biswick Mwale, head of Malawi's National AIDS Commission

Public failures:
Unaffordable and unavailable medicines

- India is the world's primary source of affordable anti-retroviral medicines used to treat HIV.
- Of 1,556 new medicines produced by the multinational pharmaceutical industry between 1975–2004, only 21 medicines addressed the diseases that primarily affect poor people in developing countries.
- Two million die every year of TB, and yet there are not enough new medicines to treat and reverse the spread of TB.

Unaffordable medicines

Access to affordable, quality medicines is critical for patients in poor countries who suffer from a disproportionately high burden of disease – and for their governments, for whom the cost of medicine is a large component of their national health-care budgets.

Many poor people pay for medicines themselves. The high prices mean that patients must either skip treatment or choose between medicines and other basic necessities. Women suffer a greater burden because of their role as caretakers of sick family members and as income earners. Women are also the last to seek medical attention when cost is involved.

Patents vs. Patients

WTO (World Trade Organisation) intellectual property rules established under the TRIPS (Trade Related Aspects of Intellectual Property Rights) Agreement created 20-year monopolies for medicines in developing countries, keeping prices high by preventing the introduction of inexpensive, generic versions. Under the TRIPS Agreement, developing countries are empowered to use basic safeguards to reduce the price of medicines to protect public health. Yet rich countries and the pharmaceutical industry have fought any attempt to do so. This led to public outrage, and Oxfam joined with others to campaign to cut the cost of medicines in poor countries. In a landmark victory, the campaign helped stop 39 pharmaceutical companies from taking the South

African government to court over its laws to reduce prices. Public pressure also led to the 2001 'Doha Declaration': members of the WTO agreed that intellectual property rules would no longer obstruct developing countries' efforts to protect public health.

More than two million people living with HIV and AIDS in low- and middle-income countries were receiving treatment in 2006, a 54 per cent increase from the previous year. Generic competition was an important factor in the reduction of the price of first-line anti-retroviral medicines from US$10,000 per patient per year to only US$100 per patient per year.

Unavailable medicines

Millions in the developing world continue to suffer from HIV and AIDS, TB, and malaria. Children still die of chest infections and diarrhoea. And non-communicable diseases, such as heart disease, asthma, cancer, and cardiovascular disease are imposing a double burden upon poor people.

Diseases which primarily affect poor people in developing countries remain untreated, because few medicines have been developed by the multinational pharmaceutical industry over the last three decades. Strict intellectual property rules do not create incentives for drug companies to develop medicines to treat these diseases, because poor people are not an attractive market for the pharmaceutical industry.

"I am worried because voices like mine are not counted by anyone. I do not have any idea how many people like me have started counting down the days," says Umashankar, a 35-year-old father of five who is HIV positive. He is one of millions of people across India unable to afford the more expensive anti-retroviral medicines he needs. Hundreds of thousands of poor people could be saved if their health were put before drug company profits.

- Patented medicines continue to be priced out of reach for most people in developing countries.
- Some countries have tried to undermine the Doha Declaration by imposing ever-stricter levels of intellectual property protection on behalf of pharmaceutical companies.
- Trade rules pushed by rich countries and pharmaceutical companies remain a major barrier to accessing affordable versions of patented medicines.
- Neglected diseases continue to afflict millions of poor people in developing countries, and there are scarcely any new medicines to treat these diseases.
- Even though donors and national governments have pledged significant additional funds for global health, the high cost of medicines could undermine the benefits of this extra money.
- Although the price of the older first-line anti-retroviral medicines (ARVs) has been reduced, patented second-line ARVs are approximately 15 times the cost of generic first-line medicines and are still unaffordable for many public and private treatment programmes.
- New medicines that can effectively treat non-communicable diseases are unaffordable to most people in developing countries and for those governments committed to provide universal access to medicines.

This is Nana Diasamidze.
She's a health-care adviser in Batumi, Georgia.

It's a complicated job, but to put it simply, she spends her time working to get health care for people who otherwise wouldn't be able to afford it. "I'm driven by the desire to help and represent poor people," she says. "It's essential that the government expands the range of medical services it provides, so everyone can access quality health care. Healthy people make a healthy country."

The Georgian government has recently begun to prioritise privatisation in the health sector. Some estimates suggest that as many as 52 per cent of the population lives in poverty, meaning that the new privatised system will leave many people unable to afford medical care.

As a health ombudswoman working for local organisation Step Forward, Nana monitors people's access to care in Batumi and the surrounding villages. "I help to protect, and advocate for, the rights of medical patients," she explains. "I provide people with information and advice on their rights and on the benefits available to them. I tell them about existing local and national health programmes. And I give out information, and advocate for change."

Having spoken to people who are missing out on basic health care, Nana is convinced that the new system has to change. "The government needs to improve and modify state assistance to include families who do not presently qualify for it but are genuinely in need."

The current situation shows some of the problems that can arise when free, good quality health care is not available to everyone. Nana shakes her head as she tells stories of people missing out on state treatment because they were unable to pay, but she remains totally committed to her role. "I love my job and the work I do," she says. "Every day that I am in a position to help people in need is a happy day."

GEORGIA PROFILE

- Georgia is a middle-income country but has seen a severe deterioration in public investment in health and education since independence: the government spends just one per cent of its gross domestic product (GDP) on health and 2.9 per cent on education. This is far less compared with other countries in the region, which have had similar histories.

- 52 per cent of the population lives below the national poverty line.

- 12.6 per cent of the population is unemployed (World Bank) but some civil-society organisations estimate that unemployment rates have reached 35 per cent in towns and 60 per cent in rural areas.

ONE PERSON CAN MAKE A BIG DIFFERENCE.
IMAGINE WHAT SIX MILLION CAN DO.

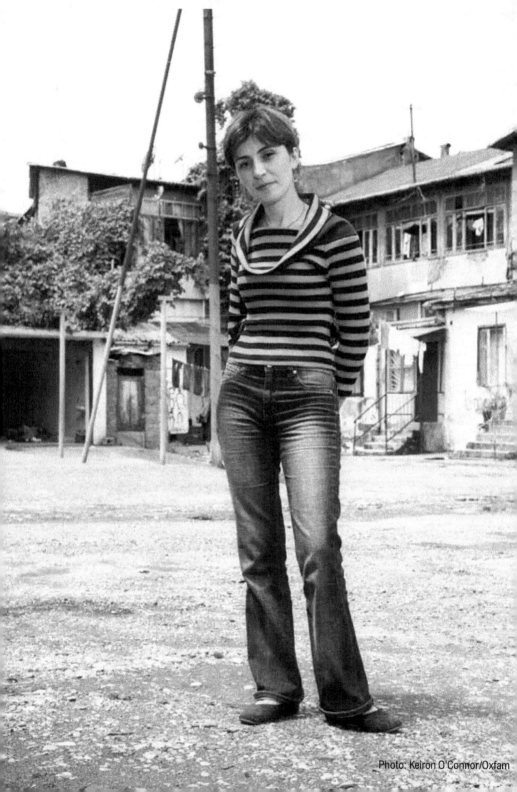

Photo: Keiron O'Connor/Oxfam

Public failures:
Unco-ordinated and fragmented services

The contribution of civil society

When governments fail to provide services, most poor people get no education, health care, clean water, or sanitation. Those who do either have to bankrupt themselves to pay for private services, or rely on civil-society providers such as mosques, churches, charities, and community groups.

Informal provision of health care and education through local organisations is common in many countries. Although they can pioneer innovative approaches to service provision, and support citizens in claiming their rights to health, education, and water, their coverage is partial, services are hard to scale up, and the quality can vary greatly.

Evidence shows that citizens' initiatives work best when integrated into a publicly led system, with their contribution recognised and supported by government. For example, in Kerala state in India, and in Malaysia and Barbados, governments have helped to fund church schools, and have regularly monitored them to maintain standards.

The private sector

Faced with failing government services, many turn to the private sector. But private providers:
- provide their services only to the lucky few who can afford to pay
- are hard to regulate
- steal staff from the public sector
- can have a negative impact on the poorest and most vulnerable communities.

Water privatisation is the most notorious example, but under-regulated private-sector involvement in health care in developing countries is also spreading rapidly.

- When China phased out free public health, household health costs rose forty-fold and progress on tackling infant mortality slowed. Services are paid for through health insurance, which covers only one-in-five people in rural areas.

- The Georgian government has recently begun to prioritise privatisation in the health sector. Some estimates suggest that as many as 35 per cent of the population lives in poverty, meaning that the new privatised system will leave many people unable to afford medical care.

- Regulating private providers, especially multinational companies, can be more difficult for states than providing services themselves. The global water market is dominated by a few US, French, and UK companies, such as Bechtel, Suez, and Biwater: the contracts they negotiate often require guaranteed profit margins. If governments try to terminate these contracts, they risk being sued, as in the cases of Tanzania and Bolivia.

Public failures:
Rich countries – pushing the private sector

Rich-country governments and international institutions such as the World Bank can have a major influence on poor countries. Advice from outside experts, funded by aid, can help determine the reforms that a government adopts.

But instead of helping to build public services, rich-country governments and agencies often push private-sector alternatives to public-service failures:

- The World Bank and IMF still often use their influence to insist that governments introduce privatisation and increase private service provision in return for aid or debt cancellation.
- The WTO and bilateral/regional 'Free Trade Agreements' also threaten public services by limiting how governments regulate foreign service providers.
- The IMF sets arbitrary ceilings on government spending, including on teachers and health workers.

At the same time, rich countries are simultaneously urging poor countries to meet the MDGs, while aggravating skills shortages by proactively recruiting thousands of their key workers.
- Of the 489 nursing students who graduated from the Ghana Medical School between 1986 and 1995, 61 per cent have left Ghana, with more than half of them going to the UK and one-third to the USA.

...and failing to deliver

Not only are rich countries often pushing the wrong solutions, they are also failing to deliver on their aid commitments, and to ensure that debt relief is given to all countries that need it.

Despite rich countries promising in 2005 to deliver US$50 billion per year by 2010, aid levels fell in 2006. If current trends continue Oxfam estimates that rich countries will miss their target by a staggering $30 billion. At $103 billion, aid represents just ten per cent of global military spending and just 0.3 per cent of rich countries' income. This is less than half of the 0.7 per cent target they signed up to in 1970.

In 2005, rich countries also agreed to provide debt cancellation to some of the world's most highly indebted poor countries. Twenty-four countries have benefited so far, but 17 are still waiting. An additional 19 poor countries that desperately need debt cancellation have

Zambia – reaping the benefits of cancelled debts
Zambia introduced free health care for people living in rural areas for the first time in April 2006, scrapping fees which for years put health care beyond the reach of millions living in poverty. This dramatic move was the direct result of debt cancellation and aid increases agreed at the G8 in July 2005. Zambia received $4 billion in debt relief – releasing money that is now being poured directly into health and education. Extra spending on education will include funds to recruit more than 4,500 teachers, and to construct and rehabilitate schools in rural and urban areas.

been left out of the deal altogether. Poor-country governments not only need more aid, they also need aid that is well co-ordinated, predictable, and channelled through national budgets to support public systems. But what they typically get is short-term, unpredictable aid, disbursed through a jumble of different projects that often directly compete with public services for scarce resources and staff.

- Only eight cents in the aid dollar are channelled into government plans that include the training and salaries of teachers and health workers.
- As much as 70 per cent of aid for education globally is spent on 'technical assistance', much of it to highly paid consultants from rich countries.
- More than four-fifths of 35,000 aid transactions that take place each year are worth less than $1 million, and require 2,400 quarterly progress reports, according to the UK Secretary of State for International Development.
- Aid is extremely unpredictable. In 2005, Zambia was promised US$930 million in aid, but at the end of the year, rich countries only gave US$696 million – nearly one-third less.
- In health, donor demands for numerous different 'vertical' (disease specific) initiatives waste officials' time, duplicate services, and distort health priorities. Angola and the Democratic Republic of Congo, for instance, have each been required to set up four separate HIV and AIDS 'co-ordinating' bodies.

What needs to happen

Shift the political agenda

Poor-country governments must show leadership in delivering essential services for all. They should spend more on these vital services – and spend it better. And to make this happen, civil society must pile on the pressure.

Across the world, activists are doing this: getting debates on essential services into the newspapers and onto politicians' lists of priorities.

- In Kenya, the national coalition of education groups, Elimu Yetu (Our Education) played a pivotal role in making free primary education a central election issue, ensuring it was introduced in 2003; the result was that 1.2 million children went to school for the first time.

- In 2005, the world's biggest ever anti-poverty coalition was formed, the Global Call to Action against Poverty (GCAP). Last year, in the space of just one day, 24 million people in more than 80 countries stood up symbolically against poverty. Its key demands include quality universal public services for all.

- In January 2007, civil-society coalitions launched the *9 is Mine* campaign to pressure the Indian government to invest six per cent of GDP in education and three per cent in health. The campaign mobilised hundreds of thousands of children from across 14 states of India to sign a petition. India spends less on social services than Uganda, a scandal in a country that prides itself on strong economic growth and that does not rely heavily on external aid.

Poor-country governments need to:
- rapidly expand the public provision of essential services
- make sustained investments in education, health, water and sanitation services, emphasising preventative reproductive health policies, and combating HIV and AIDS
- work with civil society and the private sector within a single, integrated public system
- set a timetable for reaching the target of investing at least 20 per cent of government budgets in education and 15 per cent in health
- ensure citizen representation in monitoring public services, and involve civil society in local and national planning and budget processes, including agreements and contracts signed with donors, the World Bank, and the IMF
- take a public stand and act against corruption, prosecuting theft whenever it occurs.

Civil society needs to:
- act together to demand quality public services, including free health care and education, and subsidised water and sanitation services
- continue to build worldwide popular movements that demand government action, such as the Global Campaign for Education and the Global Call to Action against Poverty
- engage in local and national planning processes
- work with national parliaments to monitor budget spending – and ensure that services reach the poorest people, and that corruption is not tolerated
- challenge rich-country governments, the World Bank, and IMF when they fail to support public services
- work with governments and other non-state providers to ensure increased innovation, learning, co-operation, and accountability in the provision of essential services.

What needs to happen

Win the fight against corruption

Oxfam's experience from working in more than 100 countries does not support the view that all aid is misused or wasted through corruption.

Many governments are working hard to fight corruption and improve financial management, although there is a long way to go in many instances. A recent survey by the IMF of countries receiving debt relief found that spending on tackling poverty in those countries has increased by 33 per cent since 2002, which is ultimately the greatest test of whether money is reaching the poorest.

Aid can also play a key role in fighting corruption. It can:
- pay to train lawyers
- support the free press
- increase salaries of the police and other public-sector workers.

In short, aid can help build the only long-term answer to corruption: effective public services and strong democratic institutions, supported by active and informed citizens who refuse to tolerate dishonest gain.

Citizens of poor countries themselves can also play a key role in fighting corruption. Oxfam funds partners all over the world to fight corruption:
- The SEND foundation in Ghana runs monitoring committees made up of citizens in poor northern districts. They ensure that money from debt cancellation is spent effectively and is not lost through corruption.

- The Civil Society for Poverty Reduction (CSPR) in Zambia monitors the use of aid funds by the Zambian government.
- A national network of education organisations in Malawi works closely with the Parliamentary finance committee to monitor government budget commitments to education over the last three years.

But the G8 and other rich countries must also do more to tackle the 'supply side' of corruption: the export credit agencies, companies, and individuals from their own countries, who either pay or tacitly tolerate the paying of bribes.

Tackle the workforce crisis

All successful countries have built an ethos of public service, in which public-sector workers are encouraged to take pride in their contribution to the nation. Society in turn is urged to grant them status and respect.
- Pay on its own does not always increase motivation, but it is the first priority where earnings are currently too low.
- Better pay needs to be matched with better conditions. Housing is a major issue for most teachers, especially women teachers in rural areas.
- Governments must work with trade unions to achieve improved pay and conditions, combining them with codes of conduct to ensure that workers do their jobs.

Drastically scaling up the numbers of teachers and health workers is a huge task that requires strategic, co-ordinated planning between poor-country governments and aid donors. Governments must invest in competent managers and planners to produce and implement clearly costed plans.

"I have been a nurse for 30 years, and every day I see health situations that make my heart break. I see rows of newborn babies sleeping three to a baby-cot, and mothers sleeping on the floors of the district hospitals, because of lack of proper facilities. I see the hollowness in the eyes of a nurse who is starved of sleep, as she works on her third 24-hour shift in a row, to try and earn money to support her family. I see pregnant women and their unborn children exposed to HIV and AIDS, because clinics and hospitals don't have the facilities, staff, or medicines to test and treat the disease. When you become a nurse, you work in spite of these things," says Dorothy Ngoma, Director of the National Organisation of Malawian Nurses and Midwives.

Although there is still a long way to go, the situation in Malawi has slightly improved. The Malawi government has been working with the UK and other countries to co-ordinate the funding and different programmes that exist to improve Malawi's health service. The benefits are clear. In the past year, the salaries of nurses and doctors have increased by 52 per cent. The government is also planning to double the number of nurse and midwife technicians.

Make services work for women

Investing in basic services that support and empower women and girls means promoting women as workers, supporting them as service users, protecting them from abuse, and combining these measures with legal reforms that improve the status and autonomy of women in society.

In Botswana, Mauritius, Sri Lanka, Costa Rica, and Cuba, the high proportion of women among teachers and health workers has been instrumental in encouraging women and girls to use the services.

Progress is often achieved by simultaneously working with women's groups, changing laws, and challenging harmful beliefs.

In Brazil, women's organisations working within and outside government ensured that the 1988 Constitution reflected the importance of women's reproductive health, and women's movements have continued to influence public-health policy in Brazil.

Developing-country governments must:
- abolish fees for basic education and health care, and subsidise water for poor people
- make services work for women and girls, and improve their social status
- train, recruit, and retain desperately needed health workers and teachers
- set salaries of existing health workers and teachers at dignified levels, in collaboration with their unions
- build an ethos of public service, in which both public and essential service workers are encouraged to take pride in their contribution.

What needs to happen

Provide access to afforable medicines

Rich countries should:
- stop imposing stricter levels of intellectual property protection upon developing countries, and not pressure developing countries to stop using basic public-health safeguards
- provide adequate investment for research and development (R&D) into neglected diseases and developing medicines outside of the intellectual property system.

International institutions, such as WHO, should:
- support and promote the use of public-health safeguards under the TRIPS Agreement, and work closely with developing countries to develop new mechanisms that promote innovation of appropriate medicines and vaccines.

The pharmaceutical industry needs to:
- ensure access to medicines is incorporated into its core business model, and change its approach to pricing, intellectual property, and R&D to make medicines more affordable in developing countries.

Poor countries need to:
- employ public-health safeguards under the TRIPS Agreement to reduce medicine prices, and refuse to introduce stricter levels of intellectual property protection
- prioritise R&D so that it accurately reflects the actual health needs of their citizens, tackling neglected diseases and developing medicines outside the intellectual property system.

Support – not undermine – essential services

Rich countries, the World Bank, and the IMF should:

Stop pushing failed policies
- stop pushing private-sector initiatives that do not benefit poor people and, instead, support proven public-sector solutions
- stop attaching economic policy conditions to their aid and arbitrary ceilings on government spending.

Give more aid
- give 0.7 per cent of their national income as aid and allocate at least 20 per cent of that aid to basic services
- fully finance the Global Fund to Fight AIDS, TB and Malaria, and the Education for All Fast Track Initiative, ensuring that they support governments and public systems
- extend debt cancellation to all countries that are unable to reach the MDGs under their debt burden.

Give better aid
- ensure aid is co-ordinated around national plans, predictable, and directed to those people who need it most
- give as much as possible of their aid in the form of long-term general or sector budget support.

Support policies that work
- support the expansion of publicly provided essential services
- support the removal of user fees in basic health care and education, and subsidise water fees for poor people
- work with poor countries to recruit, train, and retain 4.25 million new health workers and 1.9 million teachers, and invest in the skills of public utility/local government staff working in water and sanitation services
- end the active recruitment of health and other professionals from poor countries.

Aid can work:
UK Aid Delivers Results in Tanzania
The UK government's long-term commitment to provide aid directly to the Tanzanian government, in the face of critics, is delivering results. Budget support, aid that goes directly to the government of poor countries, has enabled the Tanzanian government to masively invest in public services. It has doubled its education budget and substantially increased its health spending. And the results for Tanzania's poor people have been impressive: for example, between 2000–2005, aid helped to reduce infant mortality by a third and under-5 mortality by a quarter.

Aid can work:
Kenya Reduces Child Deaths From Malaria
The number of children dying from malaria has dropped sharply in areas of Kenya, where the disease is endemic, as a result of a campaign to provide free insecticide-treated mosquito nets to families. This campaign was funded with money from the Global Fund to Fight AIDS, TB and Malaria, and from the UK government.

According to the World Health Organisation, there was a near ten-fold increase in the number of young children sleeping under insecticide-treated mosquito nets between 2004 and 2006 in targeted districts, resulting in a reduction of malaria-related deaths by 44 per cent.

Conclusion

Within a generation, for the first time in history:
- every child in the world could be in school
- every woman could give birth with the best possible chance that neither she nor her baby would die
- everyone could drink water without risking their lives
- millions of new health workers and teachers could be saving lives and shaping minds
- everyone could have access to affordable, quality medicine.

We know how to achieve this – political leadership, government action, and public services, supported by long-term flexible aid from rich countries and debt cancellation.

We know that the market alone cannot do this. Civil society can pick up some of the pieces, but governments must act. There is no short cut, and no other way.

To achieve these goals, developing-country governments must fulfil their responsibilities, their citizens must pressure them to do so, and rich countries must support and not undermine them. And rich countries must deliver what they have promised.

Essential services – health, education, water and sanitation – could transform the lives of millions of poor people and are the key to making poverty history.

For the full report, *In the Public Interest,* and for sources visit: **www.oxfam.org/forall**

"LIKE SLAVERY AND APARTHEID, POVERTY IS NOT NATURAL. IT IS MAN-MADE AND IT CAN BE OVERCOME AND ERADICATED BY THE ACTIONS OF HUMAN BEINGS."

NELSON MANDELA, 2005

THE WORLD NEEDS QUALITY HEALTH CARE AND EDUCATION...

Every day in developing countries, teachers, doctors, and nurses are changing people's lives. They work against the odds to provide quality education and decent health care – despite poor pay and lack of equipment and materials.

BUT THE WORLD NEEDS SIX MILLION MORE TEACHERS AND HEALTH WORKERS...

To enable the 80 million children who still don't go to school to get an education, and to stop the needless deaths of the 1,400 women every day in child-birth.

To make this happen, we have to put pressure on governments.

WE NEED SIX MILLION OF YOU TO PLEDGE YOUR SUPPORT...

Join the growing global movement that's demanding health and education for all.

HEALTH&EDUCATION
FOR ALL

Building strong public services could transform the lives of millions of people – and, with political leadership, it is well within the grasp of our generation.

This booklet has all you need to know about the role of public services in developing countries, and their role in making poverty history.

It has information on how governments, civil-society organisations, private companies, international donors, and the World Bank and International Monetary Fund, must change the way they act to guarantee health and education for all.

© Oxfam International 2008

www.oxfam.org/forall

Oxfam International is a confederation of thirteen development agencies working together in more than 100 countries to find lasting solutions to poverty and suffering: Oxfam America, Oxfam-in-Belgium, Oxfam Canada, Oxfam France - Agir Ici, Oxfam Australia, Oxfam GB, Oxfam Hong Kong, Intermón Oxfam (Spain), Oxfam Ireland, Oxfam Novib (Netherlands), Oxfam New Zealand, Oxfam Quebec, and Oxfam Germany.

The international NGO dedicated exclusively to the provision of safe domestic water, sanitation and hygiene education to the world's poorest people.

Charity registration number 288701

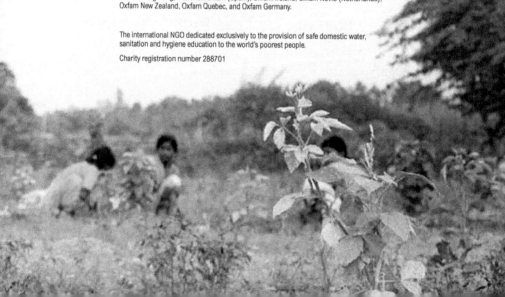

Printed in the USA
CPSIA information can be obtained
at www.ICGtesting.com
JSHW012013140824
68134JS00024B/2397